Natural Weight Loss

Health & Fitness

The Smart & Easy Guide to Naturally Healthy

By Marguerite Fuscia

www.BeachChairFitness.com

M@BeachChairFitness.com

800-738-9464

ISBN-10: 0615837751
ISBN-13: 978-0615837758 - Beach Chair Fitness Publishing

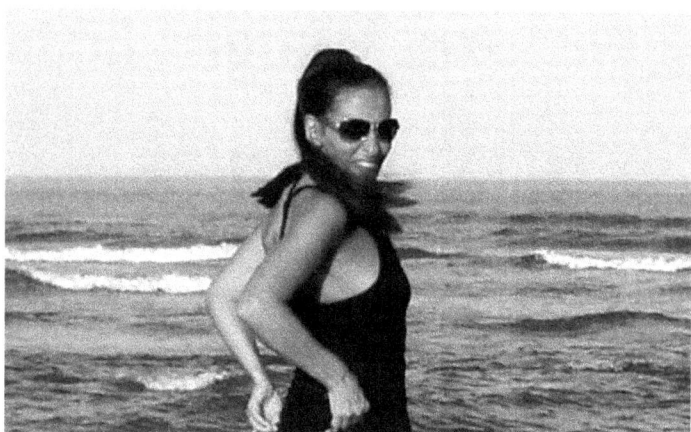
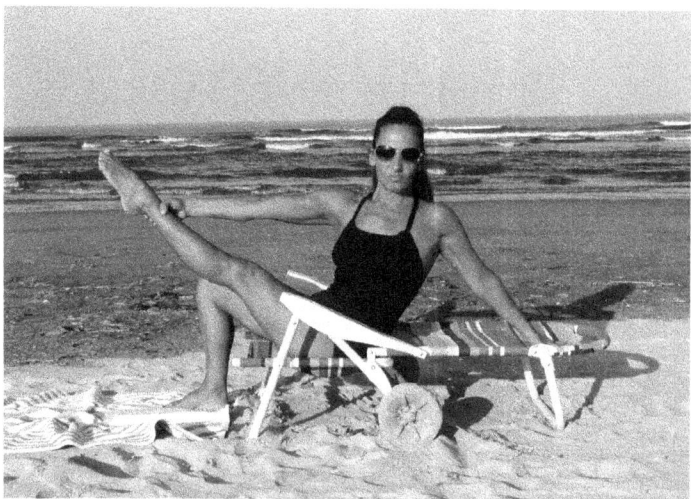

DEDICATION

This book is dedicated to all the people who are willing to help themselves, as that gives them the opportunity to help others.

ACKNOWLEDGMENTS

I would like to acknowledge the following people for their inspiration and assisting me in creating this book:
Joyce Meyer, Louise Hay, John my Yoga Master, all the people that come to my classes and my Family.

Required Disclaimer

About the Author

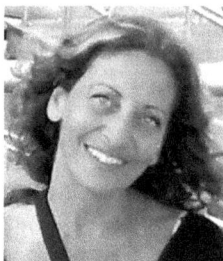

Marguerite Fuscia combined her love for fitness with her love of the beach to create the Beach Chair Fitness platform.

The proprietary Beach Chair Fitness Programs show people of all ages and fitness levels how to derive health and a fun and effective full body workout in virtually any indoor or outdoor setting. The core concepts are rooted in common sense, practical application and saving people time. Marguerite imparts a simple to follow diet and nutrition guide and valuable tips for living a healthful lifestyle. Her direct and balanced teaching style appeals to fitness lovers of all ages.

Marguerite understands the importance of being able to teach effectively to groups of children, men and women of mixed ages.
Her natural teaching ability emerged at a young age. When she was only 14 years old, she was recruited by her dance instructors to teach Jazz classes. Certified in Fitness, Health, Nutrition and Yoga, she has had extensive anxiety and stress management training and is a lifetime member of Weight Watchers. In her early days in the mid 1990's, Marguerite was one of the first to implement the "Boot Camp" workout style into her personal daily regimen while living in Fort Lauderdale, Florida. Marguerite introduced her signature brand of fitness applications to the City of North Wildwood, and launched their first Yoga and Boot Camp programs, which are flourishing.

For more information, consultation or to book time with Marguerite, please send her an email directly at Marguerite@BeachChairFitness.com or call 800-738-9464.

Table of Contents

Dedication   2

Acknowledgments   3

Required Disclaimer   4

About The Author   5

Introduction   11

1 Stay Hydrated   14

2 Your Mom was Right, NEVER Skip Breakfast   14

3 Get Your Omega 3 Daily   16

4 Work up a Sweat   16

5 Add Variety to Your Exercise Routine   18

6 Get Enough Sleep   18

7 Enjoy Mind and Body Exercises   19

8 Learn and Employ Relaxation Techniques   20

9 Ditch Processed Foods for Healthier Snack Options   21

10 Discover the Healthy Goodness of Green Tea   22

11 Take Food Supplements   22

12 Wash Your Hands Often   23

13 Phase Out Unhealthy Vices   25

14 Take Annual Health Tests   25

15 Be Kind to Yourself   26

16 Stay Motivated   26

17 Drink Alcohol in Moderation   27

18 Limit Sugar in Your Diet as Much as Possible   28

19 Eat Complex Carbohydrates   30

20 Cut Down on Your Caffeine   31

21 Push Yourself   32

22 Take it from Nike, JUST DO IT!   32

23 Watch What You Put In Your Grocery Cart   33

24 Eat 5 to 6 Meals a Day   33

25 Eat at Home   34

26 Incorporate Physical Activities in Your Daily Life   35

27 Be Selective of Shows you Watch on TV   35

28 Make Smart Food Choices   36

29 Maintain at Least One Hobby   37

30 Bask in Love   37

31 Go Organic   38

32 Avoid Negative People and Situations   38

33 Explore   39

34 Don't Confuse Thirst with Hunger   40

35 Eat at a Leisurely Pace   40

36 Avoid Stress Eating   41

37 Avoid Eating while Watching TV or at the Movies   42

38 Teach Yourself to Control Cravings   43

39 Seek Support from Family and Friends   43

40 Beat Temptations Through Distraction   44

41 Keep a Diary or Journal   44

42 Remember the Importance of Emotional Fitness   45

43 Don't Over Indulge on One Thing   45

44 Find a Fitness Buddy   46

45 Ride a Bike to Work   46

46 Be Conscious with Your Food Portions   47

47 Increase Fiber in Your Daily Diet   47

48 Enjoy After Dinner Walks   48

49 Bake, Steam or Grill Instead of Frying   49

50 Avoid All-You-Can-Eat Buffets   49

51 Only Take Food Amounts You Can Comfortably Eat   50

52 Start Your Meals with Salads   51

53 Replace Sugar with Honey   52

54 Avoid Skipping Meals   52

55 Trade Baked Goodies for Fresh Fruits   53

56 When Eating Out, Choose the Healthiest Meals   53

57 Avoid Using Condiments   54

58 When Travelling, Check out Gym Facilities   55

59 When Travelling, Do Your Research and Find Local Restaurants that Offer Healthy Alternatives   56

60 Bring Your Lunch   56

61 Trade Your Desk Chair for an Exercise Ball   57

62 Use Your Break Time Wisely   57

63 Conduct a Meeting On The Go   58

64 Invest In a Pedometer   58

65 Learn to Modify   59

66 Take Vacations from Work, NOT from Good Health   59

67 Learn to Express Your Feelings   60

68 Maintain a Positive Attitude   61

69 Try Meditation   62

70 Reinforce Your Faith   63

71 Stay Young at Heart   63

72 Stay in Touch with Friends   64

73 Perform Regular Stretching Exercises   64

74 Keep Talking   65

75 Stop Smoking   65

76 Aim High   66

77 Keep Yourself Updated   67

78 Know Your Body   67

79 Go Easy on the BBQ   68

80 Treat your Brain Like a Muscle   68

81 Get Nutty   69

82 Stay Protected From The Sun   69

83 Mind Your Posture   70

84 Avoid Processed Food Products   70

85 Always Carry a Water Bottle Wherever You Go   71

86 Get Plenty of Fresh Air   72

87 Take Advantage of Natural Sunlight   72

88 Take The Stairs   73

89 Women Must visit an OBGYN Regularly   73

90 Walk and Stretch During Road Travel   74

91 Visit Your Dentist Regularly   74

92 Work Out With Kids   75

93 Substitute Walks for Emails   75

94 Warm Up Before Exercise   76

95 Take a Stand   76

96 Park Farther Away   77

97 Use Chicken Breast and Take the Skin Off   78

98 Learn to Decipher Food Labels   78

99 Check Your Cabinets   79

100 Choose to Plan Ahead   80

101 Find Healthy Alternatives   80

102 Keep Moving Forward   81

103 Raise Your Hands   81

104 Leverage The Power of Affirmations   82

105 Meditation   85

Conclusion   87

INTRODUCTION

My name is Marguerite and I'm here to help you!

IT'S A FACT...

If you want more out of life, you need to be ready to commit more and invest more into staying fit and eating right.

While there have been innumerable diet plans and exercise programs sprouting like mushrooms nowadays -- all claiming to provide the fastest results. We all know the basic equation to staying fit and healthy is the proper attitude, regular exercise and proper diet.

It has been called by many names, defined in so many ways and presented in so many forms but all health and fitness programs boil down to these three disciplines:

1. **ATTITUDE**
2. **HEALTHY EATING**
3. **REGULAR EXERCISE**

There are no other ways to approach it if you want lasting results.

Despite this common knowledge of what needs to be done to stay fit and healthy, most of us struggle not to fall off the wagon. Many still have to contend with the frustrating battle of beating the bulge.

The weight loss industry has become a highly lucrative market, with food manufacturers, nutrition experts, and plastic surgeons all feeding from the growing desperation and depression of overweight and obese people worldwide.

While the winning equation leading to fitness and health is so simple and straightforward, it remains a great challenge. The demands of daily living such as work-related stress, social pressures, life changes, holidays, travel, winter seasons, and everything else in between – are all contributing factors that can disrupt fitness routines and upset diet regimens.

The real challenge here is how to stay committed and consistent with a program despite internal and external factors that often come into play.

This book is designed to help you equip yourself with tips, tactics and practical advice on how you can stay fit and healthy today.

Success doesn't need to be a constant struggle. Fitness and healthy living is not a temporary phase or a convenient solution you can readily pull out from your closet in time for the summer season or during special occasions. If you want lasting results, ditch the 2-week plan or the 6-month program. Use common sense to make health and fitness an integral part of your lifestyle, as it should be, and you will succeed.

Read on and find out how you can live, breathe, eat, move and think healthy. I know you can do it. Do it for yourself. Start today!

To Your Continued Success,

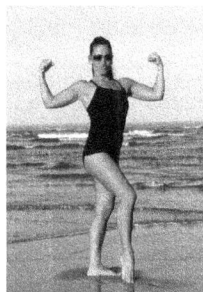

Marguerite

1

Stay Hydrated.

This is one of the most important advices you can ever get when it comes to staying healthy and fit. Drinking water every chance you get, or at least every couple of hours. Water helps ensure your body systems will keep running smoothly and it also plays a vital role in weight loss. So don't forget to drink up. I like to add some lemon into my water. I also have warm water with lemon in the morning before breakfast.

2

Your Mom was Right, NEVER Skip Breakfast.

You have probably heard it over and over how breakfast is the most important meal of the day. It really is! According to numerous medical studies, people who skip this meal actually have increased risks of gaining weight. I find that adding protein to your breakfast helps keep you fuller throughout your day. Always keep in mind to make your breakfast one of your bigger meals because you do have the rest of the day to burn off those calories. There is also that little known fact that people tend to take in higher calories all throughout the day after missing their breakfast.

Breakfast helps stabilize the body's metabolism. Ditching your first meal of the day will result to an increase in LDL levels or bad cholesterol and lower insulin levels. The increase in bad cholesterol in the body will result to clogged arteries, which can lead to a number of serious health complications such as heart disease. If you are trying to lose weight, have a small fruit, granola or yogurt for breakfast. Make sure to check the number of grams of sugar on your yogurt. The best choice is plain with fresh fruit.

3

Get Your Omega 3 Daily.

Recent studies conducted by University of Western Ontario revealed that regular intake of fish oil supplements can speed up burning of calories by as much as 400 more calories. Fish oil and Flaxseed oil supplements are rich in Omega 3, which is also effective in the prevention of the hardening of the arteries, which is one of the leading causes of heart diseases. However, it is generally best to check with your physician first before adding fish oil supplements into your daily regimen. In many cases I prefer to eat a handful of walnuts or other foods that contain omega 3, rather than a supplement.

4

Work up a Sweat.

Make exercise a part of your daily routine. Regular exercise helps keep the heart healthy. There are number of ways you can incorporate exercise into your lifestyle, so it's simply a matter of finding one that best suits you. Try to exercise at least 3 to 4 times a week, you will be surprised how many calories a simple jog or brisk walk can burn. To give you an idea, here are some examples:

• Biking at a leisurely pace for 1 hour = a total of 230 to 340 calories burned.

• Walking at a moderate pace for 1 hour = a total of 205 to 300 calories burned.

• Jogging at a moderate pace for 1 hour = a total of 300 to 600 calories burned.

• Try some exercise videos which can be done in thirty minutes and burn even more.

• Interval training works well as it allows the heart rate to rise and come back down a little. For example, run for 60 seconds, then walk for 60 seconds and repeat.

5

Add Variety to Your Exercise Routine.

Keep things light and fun by changing your fitness routine every now and then. Explore activities that aid weight loss. Go outside and jog along the park or by the beach. Consider taking up strength training, mountain climbing, cycling or other activities that can make exercise more fun and exciting. Check out some classes in your local area. I teach a boot camp that takes place right on the beach. Many years ago I started teaching Yoga classes on the beach which really provided some special experiences for myself and my students.

6

Get Enough Sleep.

With today's fast-paced lifestyle and gruelling schedules, sleep is often taken for granted. The average person needs to have 7 to 8 hours of sleep every night. If you want to maintain a healthy weight, sleep should be given equal importance, as it is the only time the body can heal and repair itself and regenerate nerve energy. Lack of sleep also impairs brain function. Try not to get too upset if you don't get eight hours, but just do your best. When you fall short, try to take a little time to rest throughout your day. A fifteen minute rest or meditation can help a lot.

7

Enjoy Mind and Body Exercises.

Consider taking yoga or tai chi classes. These exercises do not only stretch your muscles as well as strengthen the bones, sinews and joints; it can also help to teach you to relax mentally.

Mind and body exercises are wonderful way to allow oxygen to connect with your muscles and cells. Breathing exercises found in yoga oxygenate the cells. Disease can't grow in oxygenated cells. This can allow for a healthy body. It can help ease anxiety and pain as well as speed up recovery time.

8

Learn and Employ Relaxation Techniques.

It's no secret that stress contributes to weight gain and development of chronic disease. By learning relaxation responses, you can stop the adverse effects that come with stress. Among the popular relaxation techniques include breathing exercises, journaling, visualization and laughter, among others. If you deal with serious amount of stress on a daily basis, you can re-train your brain and teach your body how to best cope with it. In my experience, I firmly believe that utilizing a series of positive affirmations in your daily regimen can have a profound effect on the quality of your life. An affirmation is simply a statement of truth. Go to page --, or number 103 and start your using your affirmation exercises today. In my opinion, this is one of the most important things you can do for yourself!

9

Ditch Processed Foods for
Healthier Snack Options.

Cultivate smarter food choices to stay fit and healthy. This includes choosing your snacks with more thought and consideration. If you enjoy a bag of chips while watching TV or movie, replace it with healthier snack choices like apple slices, a small yogurt or almonds. These can satisfy your cravings minus the calories. If you want to have the chips I suggest the low sodium ones with simple ingredients. Always watch your portion size.

Keep your healthy snacks readily on hand so you won't be tempted to indulge in junk food. Make sure you don't have junk food and unhealthy food products on your desk and pantry. By keeping it out of sight, you won't feel deprived. I'll pack carrots or nuts to take on the go so I don't make bad choices.

10

Discover the Healthy Goodness of Green Tea.

Drink this Japanese staple and discover how green tea can aid in rapid weight loss. You can use it to quench your thirst instead of soda and other fizzy drinks. Green tea has been known to work well with a number of health conditions include rheumatoid arthritis, cardiovascular diseases, impaired immune function, infections, high cholesterol levels and even certain forms of cancer. Buying drinks with green tea in them may also have hidden sugar so be sure to check your labels.

11

Take Food Supplements.

If you are trying to cut down on your calorie intake, chances are, you may be also compromising your nutrition. The best way to augment the depleted vitamins and minerals in the body is through supplementation. Discuss this with your physician and determine which type of supplementation will best address you nutrition requirements. Food supplements may be a good way for extra nutrition, but always make sure to read labels and research brands. Remember that the best vitamins come from healthy food.

12

Wash Your Hands Often.

One preventive measure to avoid getting sick or contamination is by washing hands thoroughly and regularly. This may be a very basic habit that has been inculcated in us since early childhood, but one that is often overlooked. Just because your hands look clean doesn't mean they really are. Here are some guidelines on washing hands:

Wash hands before:

• Preparing meals
• Before eating

- Treating wounds
- Giving medication
- Caring for the injured and sick

Wash hands after:

- Handling food, especially when handling raw meat and poultry
- Using the toilet
- Changing diapers
- Touching toys, pets and waste
- Coughing, blowing of nose, and sneezing into hands
- Treating wounds
- Caring for the injured and sick
- Handling chemicals and garbage or anything that might be contaminated

It's always a good idea to carry an antibacterial lotion or spray to use in a pinch, but it won't replace a good hand washing.

13

Phase Out Unhealthy Vices.

Cultivate healthy habits and get rid of the ones that pose adverse effects on your health. Anything in excess can be bad and you don't want your health to suffer the consequences.

Almost everyone has some negative health habits. It's OK! You don't need to beat yourself up, just try to change them a little at a time. A small one percent change implemented consistently over time can really add up. This can make things less stressful.

14

Take Annual Health Tests.

Annual physical examinations are generally covered by health insurance or you can also get one for free or at a minimal cost. Routine tests are critically important to detect health problems at an early stage before they grow into a serious health issue.

15

Be Kind to Yourself.

Treat yourself every now and then! This can consist of a simple pampering such as getting your hair done at a posh salon, or scheduling a massage appointment. Break away from the demands and pressures of daily living and allow yourself to slow down, recharge and find temporary relief. Taking a warm bath with candles can do the trick if money is tight, but always take time for yourself.

16

Stay Motivated.

It can be a real challenge to stay on track to a health and fitness program if you are no longer motivated. Seek inspiration. Find ways to stay motivated to make smarter choices and proper decisions every single day. You are constantly faced with choices that pose real temptations such as choosing between watching TV and working out, or choosing between a chocolate chip cookie and a piece of fruit. Starting a routine that makes you feel good like exercise will automatically become a habit you won't want to miss. Remember even a fifteen minute routine will help. It goes by quicker than you think. Try to keep people that motivate you on your speed dial for help in a pinch.

17
Drink Alcohol in Moderation.

Alcohol shows up at almost every social event, especially during the holiday season. Learn to limit your intake to no more than one or two drinks since too much alcohol can disrupt your sleep and make you feel sluggish the following day, not to mention contribute to extra calories. It's important to choose drinks without a lot of sugary content. For example, choose a vodka and club instead of fruity juices or soda mix. Get drinks on the rocks, since the ice adds extra water. Have a glass of water in-between your cocktails.

18

Limit Sugar in Your Diet as Much as Possible.

We all know that sugar can be detrimental to your health. The problem is it's a staple and included in so many products we see every day. Make sure to read the labels and learn to steer clear from any processed food products as it is most likely laden with too much sugar. Nutrition experts recommend limiting added sugar to no more than 10 tablespoons a day. Sugar substitutes are really not a good way to go.

However, sugar can come in so many forms and under many names. Be extra wary on food products that contain the following:

- Glucose
- High fructose corn syrup
- Lactose
- Honey
- Fruit juice concentrates
- Molasses
- Maltose

- Sucrose / Sucralose
- Brown sugar
- Fructose

To give you an idea on the sugar content on some of the popular food products and beverages, refer to the data provided below:

- Regular soda   33%
- Candies   16%
- Cakes, pies and cookies   13%
- Fruit drinks   10%

Individuals who are constantly exposed to consumption of food products with high sugar content also increase their calorie intake and lower micronutrient supply. Again, remember to read those labels...

19

Eat Complex Carbohydrates.

When it comes to losing weight and eating right, we all know we need to watch our carb intake. However, there are good carbohydrate sources that are perfectly safe to eat. However, you need to closely monitor the sources of your carbohydrates as there is a huge difference between complex and simple carbohydrates.

Simple carbohydrates contain high amounts of sugar that need to be broken down by the body. While this type of sugar provides energy, when not assimilated, gets converted to fat. This is the reason why many diets restrict the intake of carbohydrate-rich food. Simple carbohydrates can contribute to weight gain and are especially risky for pregnant women.

On the other hand, complex carbohydrates, while containing sugar also feature more complex chains, making it more difficult to break it down. This allows the human body ample time to use it longer. Another great benefit of complex carbs is the high fiber content, which add bulk to the diet, effectively warding off hunger and at the same time alleviates and prevents constipation.

Some simple carbohydrate food sources are: Table sugar, brown sugar, corn syrup, honey, maple syrup, molasses, jams, jellies, fruit drinks, soft drinks and candy.

Here are some excellent sources of complex carbohydrates: Green vegetables, whole grains and foods made from them, such as oatmeal, pasta, and whole-grain breads, starchy vegetables such as potatoes, sweet potatoes, corn, pumpkin, beans, lentils, and peas.

20

Cut Down on Your Caffeine.

Too much caffeine can be bad for your health. Limit your intake to at least one to two cups per day. However, a lot of people are actually silent victims of caffeine addiction with common symptoms that include irritability, anxiety, upset stomach, poor concentration, insomnia, and depression, among others. I find it better to grind whole beans when making coffee. If you buy it when you're out, most of the best coffee is found in coffee shops, where you can see them making it with whole beans. It is usually stronger so you won't need that twenty four ounce.

21

Push Yourself.

You've probably heard advice telling you not to be so hard on yourself. There is a huge difference between castigating yourself and adhering to self-discipline. You can push yourself in a positive way! Don't allow self-imposed pressure overwhelm you instead of motivate you. Using affirmation exercises can help you stay in a positive mind-set.

22

Take it from Nike, JUST DO IT!

Most times we find ourselves willing victims of procrastination, always putting off exercise and diet for another day. Instead of overthinking and over-planning things, just go ahead and do it. You will soon find your momentum and discover that the hardest part is simply getting started. Taking small steps toward better health is a fantastic way to start. Apply new elements every once in a while so the change becomes the norm and therefore easier to follow.

23
Watch What You Put In Your Grocery Cart.

One cardinal rule you need to vigilantly follow is to never do your grocery shopping on an empty stomach. Otherwise, you will find yourself falling prey to compulsive buying. Instead, prepare a complete list of the things you need and make sure not to deviate from it. Stick to whole, fresh food products. Filling your cart with whole foods is always a good idea. If you want a snack, there are some good choices. Implement "Perimeter Shopping", meaning buying mainly from the areas on the outer walls of the store. Most supermarkets are organized in this manner. Read the labels. Make sure the ingredients are readable and not filled with a lot of chemicals and sugar.

24

Eat 5 to 6 Meals a Day.

Many people who go on a diet often complain about dealing with hunger pangs and that nagging sense of deprivation. One way to combat this is to replace your 3 large meals with 5 to 6 small ones. Sounds good right? Just eat small portions and you'll be set. This will prevent you from overeating and caving in to temptation. Regular food intake can pump up your metabolism.

25

Eat at Home.

One major factor that contributes to weight gain is the propensity to eat fast food meals, processed foods, takeout and microwave dinners – all of which are heavily laden with calories. While it may require some extra time and effort to prepare meals from scratch, you should never compromise your health for convenience. There are tons of delicious, quick no-fuss recipes you can use to whip up meals in minutes.

26

Incorporate Physical Activities in Your Daily Life.

Maximize every chance you get to move your body and work out. You don't really need to go to the gym to burn calories. There are so many ways you can pump up your metabolism by making simple changes, such as taking the stairs instead of the elevator and parking father away so you will be forced walk the rest of the way. Play with your kids, stretch and perform push ups during commercial breaks. Do everything you can to stay active all throughout the day. Remember, these are good additional examples. Always try to do some kind of workout routine daily.

27

Be Selective of Shows you Watch on TV.

The concept here is to limit TV time before you unwittingly turn into a couch potato. If you tend to enjoy watching too much TV too often, you won't realize how much time you spend in front of the boob tube.

According to studies, too much TV can lead to early death. A sedentary lifestyle can cut years from your life and increase the risk of heart disease. While TV in itself is not harmful, being in a prolonged sitting position leads to the general absence of muscle movement, which can significantly disrupt the body's metabolism. Try to watch only the shows you really enjoy and not just zone out to anything that's on. Get up off the couch and stretch every so often.

28

Make Smart Food Choices.

Some diets impose impossible restrictions that are simply not practical and sustainable. You don't want to go on a crash diet for a specific period of time. Instead, cultivate a healthy living that will last a lifetime. This includes the small choices you make every single day. You can start by reading food labels and limit the chemical, sodium and sugar content. Slowly eliminate processed foods from your grocery bag and kitchen.

29

Maintain at Least One Hobby.

Find an activity you are passionate about that you won't mind doing for hours. You may choose landscape photography, vising museums or spending hours in a bookstore. Learn to play an instrument. Combing thrift shops for hidden treasures can prove to be very rewarding and fun. Pursue things that bring you the greatest joy.

30

Bask in Love.

If you have a significant other, family or friends, or even your pet dog, take time to connect and enjoy their company. Establish connections and nurture relationships. It can do wonders for your health and general well-being.

31

Go Organic.

You have probably heard reports on how even fresh produce today can be exposed to chemicals, pesticides and radiation. It is generally best to get your food from local, organic sources when possible. With the growing demand for such products, you can easily find different varieties and brands that are labelled organically grown or produced. However, be prepared to spend more for such products. If price or availability is an issue, make the best selections you can and remember to wash all your fruits and vegetables thoroughly.

32

Avoid Negative People and Situations.

Too much emotional stress can wreak havoc in your well-being. This does not mean you should avoid confrontations altogether. Learn to draw the lines. There's no use being around people who belittle you and undermine your goals and dreams. Prolonged exposure to stress can trigger binge eating, loss of sleep and depression, which ultimately leads to weight gain. Always try to see the positive aspects in the people around you. If they seem to make you feel stressed, then try to limit time spent around them.

33
Explore.

See a new part of the world or try out a new sport or activity. Move beyond your comfort zone every once in a while. It will do you good! Adding something new and pursuing something worthwhile will help keep you active and alive, as it breaks the usual humdrum. Open up to new experiences and be more accommodating to new changes. New experiences will lead to deeper self-discovery and a more meaningful life.

34

Don't Confuse Thirst with Hunger.

The human body has difficulty differentiating thirst from hunger. What initially seems like a food craving is actually dehydration. When you are starting to feel hunger pangs, avoid indulging in food right away and instead drink a glass of water and check if you are still hungry. If you want something with flavor, try squeezing an orange or lemon into your water.

35

Eat at a Leisurely Pace.

Enjoy your food and chew it thoroughly. It will usually take 20 minutes before you feel full so it's important not to shovel down your food, lest you overindulge. I was once told by my Yoga master, chew each piece forty times before swallowing. Make a ceremony of your meal.

A number of studies have confirmed that people who tend to eat slowly consume lesser amount of calories, enough to help you lose as much as 20 pounds per year. The brain takes time to register fullness of stomach, which means that by eating slowly, you have more time to realize you are already full.

36

Avoid Stress Eating.

Lots of us become unwitting victims to this pitfall. If you feel the need to binge, ask yourself what the trigger it. What is causing the stress? It may be from feeling a sense of loss, inadequacy, agitation or depression. Properly identify and confront your emotions instead of taking out your frustration on food. It may help to write down what you feel or engage in activities that will distract you and productively occupy your time.

Awareness is a key element in combatting emotional or stress eating. This is because a lot of people actually tend to eat more by simply not paying attention to what they put into their mouths. Eating without full awareness will lead to making poor food choices, overeating, as well as the inability to truly enjoy your food.

When you are working or lounging in the comfort of your home, avoid having food around areas that you can readily reach and eat mindlessly. Put the candy dish and cookie jar out of sight. Every time you feel urges and cravings, determine where it originates. Practice restraint instead of succumbing to temptation.

37

Avoid Eating while Watching TV or at the Movies.

Many people don't realize how much food they mindlessly consume while they are focused on a movie or favourite TV show. Avoid eating while you watch and simply enjoy the entertainment. If you really need to snack, have something healthy like carrot sticks or a piece of fruit. Microwave popcorn is not a good choice. I like to snack on popcorn that I prepare on the stove with a little olive oil and real corn kernels.

38

Teach Yourself to Control Cravings.

One of the common downfalls of any diet program is not the diet itself, but the individual's attitude towards food. Self-discipline is a very important character building trait you need to cultivate so you don't constantly cave in to temptation.

39

Seek Support from Family and Friends.

If you are following a special diet or a health regimen, let people who truly care about you know what you are into. Give them the chance to understand and make adjustments accordingly. A support group is very important to help you stay motivated and provide the affirmation and encouragement when you need it the most.

40

Beat Temptations Through Distraction.

Every time you find it overly difficult to resist temptation, keep yourself busy so you don't have to dwell on the thought. Allowing you to be lured in indulging on one cookie will most likely lead to another one. There's always something that needs to be done. Do your best to direct your focus elsewhere.

41

Keep a Diary or Journal.

A tremendous benefit is writing down your thoughts and feelings as it helps to put things in perspective. Journaling can also be a highly effective way to track your progress if you are trying to lose weight. Writing down all the foods that you eat during the day allows you to really analyse and understand what you're eating. This is one of the main components of the incredibly successful Weight Watchers program.

42

Remember the Importance of Emotional Fitness.

Your emotional well-being is as important as your physical fitness. If you ever feel the need to talk to sometime or vent, seek the company of trusted friends or family. In some cases, you may also want to consider taking therapy sessions. Don't hold it in, let it out!

43

Don't Over Indulge on One Thing.

Anything in excess can be a bad thing. Be smart in your choices and keep your food intake to a minimum whenever possible. Eat to nourish and nurture the body and not to see how much of a particular food or beverage your body can handle before it reacts negatively. Your overall well-being and health should always be given first priority.

44

Find a Fitness Buddy.

If you are an interactive people person, it may be easier to stick to a health and fitness program if you have someone who can share your journey. It can be more fun to engage in activities and try out healthy recipes with someone. Bouncing ideas off another person and motivating each other can be invaluable. Check out some clubs organizations in your area to interface with people who are already making an effort to live the healthy lifestyle.

45

Ride a Bike to Work.

If possible, you may want to consider riding a bicycle to work. It's a far healthier mode of transportation not to mention a cheaper alternative as well. If the distance between your home and work is relatively close, why not take a nice bike ride? Before you do so, make sure you take all the necessary safety precautions such as wearing a protective helmet and installing headlights.

46

Be Conscious with Your Food Portions.

You may be eating eating healthy, but you are eating too much of it, it defeats the purpose of diet. Take everything in moderation. Try to keep your meal sizes to portions that are no bigger your fist.

47

Increase Fiber in Your Daily Diet.

Fiber aids in weight loss and prevents constipation. It can also help avoid the build-up of toxins in the body, which may eventually lead to other health complications. You may already be experiencing some uncomfortable symptoms and low fiber intake may be the reason.

Following a high-fiber diet can help effectively reduce the risks of heart diseases, colon cancer, diabetes as well as diverticular diseases. It also works well in lowering the cholesterol levels. To increase fiber in the diet, here are some basic guidelines:

• Increase consumption of healthy grains and cereals – oat bran, wheat germ, whole wheat flour products, high-fiber cereals and whole wheat crackers.

• Increase consumption of beans and legumes.

• Eat more fruits and veggies like carrots and bananas.

48

Enjoy After Dinner Walks.

If you have your family or a friend around, establish the routine of enjoying quiet walks around the neighborhood. It's a great way to burn calories and bond.

According to studies, moderate intensity exercises like brisk walking can promote better weight loss. As a general rule, for you to shed a single pound, you will need to burn about 3,500 calories. A 30-minute walk helps to burn off an estimated 150 calories. Contrary to popular belief, walking after dinner will not cause muscle cramps.

49
Bake, Steam or Grill Instead of Frying.

Deep fried dishes are very high in cholesterol, so it's best to avoid it. If you really need to use cooking oil in your meals, opt for cold pressed extra virgin olive oil as it is a far healthier alternative.

50
Avoid All-You-Can-Eat Buffets.

As a rule of thumb, an all-you-can-eat buffet is one of the last places a health conscious person wants to find themselves. Of course, it's possible to stick to the salad bar area (if there is one), however, you generally don't want to put yourself in a position where it is difficult to resist temptation.

51

Only Take Food Amounts
You Can Comfortably Eat.

Only place enough food on your plate that you are willing to consume, so you can avoid over-eating. Avoid indulging in second and third helpings.

It's a good practice to take only what you need from the pan and leave the rest. Don't put the entire pot on the table. This way, you will only consume the food available on the table and if you don't get up for more, you'll avoid excessive eating. If you plan to make larger dishes, store most of it in containers and freeze. This provides you convenient food alternatives so you don't have to go out for office lunches.

52

Start Your Meals with Salads.

Before enjoying the main course, have a plate of fresh green salad. You'll still need to pay attention to your choice of dressing. This will help you feel fuller just as soon as you are ready to start with the main course.

By filling up your body with water-rich and fiber-rich food, you can effectively avoid overdoing it on the high calorie meals. Eating salads first can reduce consumption of calories by a good amount.

Homemade is going to be your best bet, using cold-pressed extra virgin olive oil, from the first pressing if possible. Add some vinegar and you're all set!

53

Replace Sugar with Honey.

Consider using organic honey instead of sugar in your beverages and baked products as a healthier option. Since the goal is to cut down on sugar consumption, honey presents a perfect alternative since honey is generally sweeter than regular table sugar, which means you'll most likely use a smaller amount.

However, be extra careful when substituting sweeteners in recipes. Honey has its own distinct flavor, which can potentially ruin your baked goodies. If you decide to use table sugar, opt for brown sugar as it is less processed and contains fewer chemicals.

54

Avoid Skipping Meals.

A lot of people seem to think that the best way to lose weight is to skip meals. This can actually have a detrimental effect as it causes fluctuations in the blood sugar levels and trigger excessive hunger which can lead to overeating. Skipping meals often increases the risk of lowering your metabolism. Stick to eating small, frequent meals.

55
Trade Baked Goodies for Fresh Fruits.

Pastries, cakes and cookies are all high in carbohydrates and sugar which can lead to extra weight gain. Instead choose a piece of apple or any other fruit in season. During special occasions it's fine to have a small bit so you don't feel deprived. There are many healthy recipes for muffins and cakes that are fun to make and taste delicious.

56
When Eating Out, Choose the Healthiest Meals.

When eating out, often you are faced with an overwhelming number of unhealthy choices. Learn the art of choosing the healthier menu options. It can also help if you share your meals with your dining companions, especially if it's an informal gathering.

57

Avoid Using Condiments.

Many types of condiments are generally bad for your health so try to avoid using them as much as possible. While condiments are known to add more flavor and aroma in food, there are those that come fully loaded with sugars, syrups and chemically synthesized sweeteners which poses serious health risks. Here are some pointers on what you can use and what to avoid:

Enjoy the following condiments:
- Mustard
- Hot sauce
- Vinegars
- Cream cheese (regular)
- Worcestershire sauce (low sodium)
- Horseradish
- Pesto
- All Natural Soy sauce with low sodium
- Sour cream (regular)

Avoid the following condiments, especially ones with "light" labels since they usually contain unhealthy additives.

- Barbecue sauce
- Teriyaki sauce
- Ketchup
- Cocktail sauce
- Regular jellies and jams

58
When Travelling, Check out Gym Facilities.

Travelling out of town or out of the country should not disrupt your regular exercise regimen. Check out the available local facilities and include exercise in your itinerary. You can also bring along a few of your own simple gym equipment items like a jump rope or an elastic band if you want to exercise in the comfort of your hotel room. It's fun to take an exercise class while you're away.

59

When Travelling, Do Your Research and Find Local Restaurants that Offer Healthy Alternatives.

When you're on the road and in an unfamiliar place it can be all too easy to eat what is convenient and readily available. To help you stick to your diet, explore healthy options within the area. It's usually a smart idea to ask the front desk for assistance.

60

Bring Your Lunch.

Instead of grabbing a quick bite at the cafeteria or a nearby fast food chain, bring along a brown bag lunch. This gives you ultimate control on what types of food you eat, how it's prepared and how much you consume. It's smart to prepare large batches of meals in advance to save you the time and stress of figuring out what you're having.

61

Trade Your Desk Chair for an Exercise Ball.

The growing trend among modern offices today is the use of exercise balls in place of ordinary office chairs. This is a perfect option for people whose work requires them to spend long hours behind the desk. Exercise balls will require you to maintain proper posture and use muscles for balance. This can be a highly beneficial passive workout for desk bound employees and work-at-homers.

62

Use Your Break Time Wisely.

Instead of taking a nap or chatting with your colleagues, maximize your break time by going out for a short walk. It can be good idea to bring along some comfy shoes that you can use. Your body will thank you for giving it the extra oxygen it craves.

63

Conduct a Meeting On The Go.

Think outside the box when planning meetings. Instead of staying cooped up in the boring conference room, maximize time by conducting your meeting outdoors or while walking towards another location. This will not only save you time, it presents a perfect excuse to stretch your legs and exercise.

64

Invest In a Pedometer.

The pedometer is a super handy small device you wear to measure the number of steps you make in a day. This will help you keep track of how much ground you're covering and serve as a reminder all throughout the day. You may be surprised at the results. Using one can be fun, even like a game. It can also be an effective tool to reach your fitness objectives even while at the office or while running errands.

65

Learn to Modify.

Every so often you may find yourself in situations where it can be a challenge to stick to your fitness routine. The trick here is to learn to adjust to situations. If you don't have dumbbells around you can use canned goods or water bottles as alternative options. Simply using the resistance of your own body can provide a fantastic workout. Learn to make use of available resources and be creative.

66

Take Vacations from Work,
NOT from Good Health.

Travelling and enjoying a holiday vacation should not be an excuse to indulge in foods and activities that are generally bad for your health. Stick to your healthy food regimen, but you can allow for small indulgences on vacation and then add some more exercise to balance it out. Extend your walk or play with the kids for a little longer. Do your best to relax and let go of food related stress when on vacation.

67

Learn to Express Your Feelings.

Let it out! Keeping your emotions bottled up, you amplify stress and increase the risk of health related problems such as heart attacks, substance abuse and depression. Define the underlying negative emotions and determine its triggers. Everything is a matter of perspective. Some express feelings not only by speaking, but through music, dance and art. Learn to embrace and express positivity in your words, actions and thoughts.

68

Maintain a Positive Attitude.

Life will not always go your way. Instead of wallowing in failure, disappointments, and resentment, learn to brush it off, let it go and move forward. Whether it's a failed relationship, a lost opportunity or an unsavory situation, choose to see the positive side of things and maintain a happy disposition. There is something to learn in practically every situation. This will help you channel your energies to the right direction and rise up to the challenges.

69

Try Meditation.

If you have 2 minutes you have time to meditate. Don't let the name bother you. This centuries old practice involves control of breathing patterns and enhancing focus. This will help you clear away mental cobwebs and maintain better perspective on situations. By learning the right breathing patterns, you will be able to provide your brain the right oxygen supply to clear away mental disturbances. There are many wonderful books and videos to explore that demonstrate many ways to meditate. Go to page 85 or number 105 for a quick, easy start.

70

Reinforce Your Faith.

Develop and seek spiritual enlightenment and focus beyond material wealth. This will help you attain lasting happiness and satisfaction which is difficult to derive from material possessions. By reinforcing your faith, you can also promote better overall health and well-being.

71

Stay Young at Heart.

Don't take everything too seriously! Maintain or rekindle your inner childlike qualities. Learn to enjoy life's simple pleasures. Laughter is the best anti-aging solution and it's available for free. A good belly laugh is also proven help boost the immune system.

72

Stay in Touch with Friends.

We are faced with the increasing popularity of online social networking websites. They should not replace your personal interactions with people around you. Indulge in regular conversations and preserve Real Life social networks by joining groups and staying in touch with friends or planning activities together.

73

Perform Regular Stretching Exercises.

Stretch it out! Stretching is the best way to work out a few kinks and aches from staying in a position for far too long, like working at a desk on your computer. You'll see how simple stretches can aid in relaxation and ease muscle tension.

74

Keep Talking.

According to research, talking at least ten minutes a day to another person can promote better brain function and enhance memory. Brief chats can actually boost brain power compared to watching TV. Another study also revealed that socially active people have longer life spans.

75

Stop Smoking.

One can't stress enough the risks and ill-effects of smoking. It limits the oxygen supply of the body and result to a host of health complications including shortened life expectancy rate. It has also been found that smoking can indirectly contribute to back pain. I feel that if you cut down it can be a big start. Don't allow anyone to tell you there is a wrong way or right way for you. Cold turkey has been proven to be one of the best ways, but it may not be right for your current situation. It's a hard habit to kick but you can do it.

Smoking also has adverse effects on people around you. Second hand smokers have been known to suffer significant increased risks of health complications that can even lead to death.   Electronic cigarettes have become increasingly popular. Some have nicotine and nicotine free models and don't contain an innumerable amount of toxic ingredients. Ultimately, you don't want to replace one bad habit with another, so make sure to be conscious in how you approach removing cigarettes from your life.

76
Aim High.

Set your weight and health goals and break them down into small milestones. Small, more frequent successes will keep you motivated and focused on achieving greater goals. Write them down on paper and place it in places where you can regularly read it, serving as a constant reminder. Post a copy on your refrigerator, work desk and computer screen.

77

Keep Yourself Updated.

Conduct regular research and stay updated on the latest health discoveries and equip yourself with the knowledge to make smart food choices. The internet provides a plethora of resources on new exercise routines, new health spas in your area, and any other health and fitness-related interests. You don't need or want to buy every new product that hits the market, but awareness of them serves to build your knowledge base.

78

Know Your Body.

Determine what factors trigger weight gain for you. Set in place the best nutrition plan for your specific body type. This will help you in making day to day decisions. There are different types of bodies, which will require different weight loss and nutrition approaches. Take time to study each one and determine which particular body type or combination of body type you actually have and plan accordingly.

79

Go Easy on the BBQ.

Compared to other dishes and food preparations, barbeques are not hygienic and may increase the risks of stomach and intestine problems and infections. Always make sure your grill is properly cleansed. Table-top, portable electric grills may also serve as a healthy and safe alternative.

80

Treat your Brain Like a Muscle.

Much like any other muscle in the body, your brain also benefits from regular exercise. Enjoy activities that present a mental challenge and conscious effort. Some excellent training examples are board games, crossword puzzles and doing things with your opposite hand.

81

Get Nutty.

Nuts are healthy snack options, which can effectively stave off food cravings. Most are good source of protein nutrition. Make sure to read the labels and choose the unsalted and roasted varieties as they are known to be free from sugars, sodium and chemicals.

82

Stay Protected From The Sun.

Remember to employ some type of sunscreen, especially during hot, humid days. Protect your skin from sun damage, which can lead to premature aging. If possible wear protective headgear when exposed to direct sunlight. Excessive exposure to harmful sun's rays can cause wrinkles, spotting and cancer. Research and read labels on your sunblock. You may opt to use a more natural lotion like Pure Shea butter.

83

Mind Your Posture.

Protect your back from unnecessary damage due to poor posture. Slouching is neither attractive nor good for your spine. Maintaining proper posture can enhance mental focus and promote better blood circulation. Turn sideways and look in a mirror to help get aligned. Yoga's Mountain pose can help.

84

Avoid Processed Food Products.

Always choose fresh, whole foods as much as possible. In general, foods that are factory packaged in boxes, bags and cans should be avoided. They have been altered in some way and are highly processed, which makes them devoid of essential nutrients and instead laden with preservatives and chemicals. Removing processed foods from your diet to the best of your ability could be one of the best things you ever do for your health.

85

Always Carry a Water Bottle
Wherever You Go.

This is one of the most practical ways you can stay fit and hydrated all throughout the day. This can effectively reduce hunger cravings, prevent you from overeating, prevent irritability, headaches and cramps and promote proper body functioning. Some prefer to drink some distilled water as well since it contains less dissolved solids. Commercially bottled cases of water are OK in a pinch, but they use very thin plastic. If possible, fill your own water bottle that is made of thick, dense plastic or glass to avoid the plastic taste.

86

Get Plenty of Fresh Air.

Revitalize your body by simply inhaling fresh air. Go outside and take deep breaths. Enclosed work spaces can reduce natural air flow, which makes you more susceptible to diseases. An oxygenated body is a healthier one! Enjoy walks with a loved one, friend or dog and breathe deeply.

87

Take Advantage of Natural Sunlight.

The health benefits of natural sunlight cannot be understated. Early morning sunlight can help boost immune system and has been known to combat depression. Open your curtains when you wake up. Watching a sunrise and basking in the most powerful exchange of energy on earth is an experience that virtually anyone can benefit from.

88

Take The Stairs.

Instead of using the elevator, use the opportunity for a quick workout by taking the stairs. Even if you use the handrail, you're still raising your heart rate more than if you were standing still.

89

Women Must visit an OBGYN Regularly.

Females 18 and above should undergo an annual physical examination and include a Pap Smear test. In addition, those in their forties and above should have mammograms along with regular breast self-examinations to ensure early detection.

90

Walk and Stretch During Road Travel.

Road trips can take a toll on your legs and back, so make sure to make frequent stops. You really need to have a chance to walk around a bit, stretch the muscles and make sure the blood is circulating properly. This will not only protect your back and help you burn calories, stretching can also help you start more alert on the road when driving. Regular stops will help you feel much better upon reaching your destination.

91

Visit Your Dentist Regularly.

Good oral hygiene is an important part of overall health and wellness. It goes beyond simply brushing your teeth and flossing daily. Be aware of the ingredients in toothpastes and mouthwashes and determine if you need to start choosing more natural alternatives. Do not ignore a toothache or mouth pain. If it persists, your body is telling you something.

Avoid further health complications from infections by allowing a professional to do his or her job and help you.

92

Work Out With Kids.

Spend the weekend or your day off with playing with kids. This is the perfect opportunity to build memories, bond and spend leisure time away from the daily stresses. Plan a park or beach outing or even a trip to the zoo. Keeping up with active toddlers and pre-schoolers can be an enjoyable burst of exercise for you.

93

Substitute Walks for Emails.

When working in an office, instead of emailing your colleague, grab this opportunity to walk over and discuss things personally instead of confining communication via email. People generally will appreciate your efforts. This will speed up the communication process and also provide you the opportunity to move your body.

94

Warm Up Before Exercise.

Launching your body into intense physical exercise with cold muscles can increase the risks of injury. In fact, many physical or sports-related injuries can be prevented through proper stretching and warm ups. Whether it's a high impact sport like basketball or a game of golf, remember the importance of properly warming up the muscles to prevent strains and sprains as well as cramping and premature fatigue.

95

Take a Stand.

You will be surprised to know that standing can burn up to 34 more calories compared to sitting down. So you can modify or ditch the standard work desk with one that features vertical adjustments. Use the higher chair when needed. When answering phones, stand up and walk around, so you can burn calories at the same time.

96

Park Farther Away.

Instead of competing for the prime parking lot spot, choose to park farther away, preferably a full block away from the office. This will give you the opportunity to walk and stretch on a daily basis. You'll also have a chance to clear your mind and focus before you walk in the front door. At the end of the day, you'll have a chance to do the same before you get behind the wheel.

THE SMART & EASY GUIDE TO NATURALLY HEALTHY

97

Use Chicken Breast and Take the Skin Off.

When cooking, work with the breast portion as it contains the most amount of white meat. Since chicken meat is so versatile, you can use it in almost any type of preparation and dish. It's the perfect source of meat protein, especially for people on a diet.

98

Learn to Decipher Food Labels.

This is one skill that will prove invaluable when making smarter food choices. It takes some time and effort to know what to look for since many labels now contain arbitrary terms like "spices" and "natural flavors" which tend to blend in to the list. Generally, the longer the list, the more cause for scrutiny. Learn to interpret and properly determine if it's a safe option or an unhealthy substitute.

99

Check Your Cabinets.

Take a survey of the cabinets inside your home, particularly under the sinks and in the laundry room. Most people are not aware of the sheer volume of chemicals that are stored out of sight. Properly dispose of any old, discolored or rusted bottles, boxes and cans. Storing different kinds of chemicals together can sometimes produce an unwanted chemical reaction. Do your research online to find the best safe alternatives when choosing cleaners, detergents and home improvement and repair items.

100

Choose to Plan Ahead.

It can be significantly easier to stick to your eating regimen if you plan ahead. Schedule the menu for the following week so you don't have to spend extra time racking your brain at the last minute on what to cook and how to prepare your food. Having a weekly menu can also effectively discourage the need to order delivery and take out. Shopping for a specific menu can also save you money since you'll be making purchases in a more targeted manner.

101

Find Healthy Alternatives.

More and more people are seeking healthier options. Many traditional dishes today can be prepared as a much healthier version. For example, you can replace regular pasta noodles with spaghetti squash. It can be very rewarding to explore your options so constantly research online. By learning ways to provide healthier alternatives, you won't feel deprived when undergoing a structured diet.

102

Keep Moving Forward.

People tend to be much more motivated when they have an aim. They normally only react when they want a certain end result. The important lesson here is to always have goals. This applies to your health and fitness and overall well-being.

103

Raise Your Hands.

Stand up and raise your both of your hands high up and stretch them out. Keep them up there. Open the palms of your hands and stretch out your fingers. Now try to frown. It doesn't work, does it? For some reason it's nearly impossible not to crack a smile when you do this.

104

Leverage The Power of Affirmations.

Below is a list of strong, positive affirmations for you to use every day. Say them out loud to yourself. You may want to say them while looking into a mirror. Say them all or specifically the ones you need the most. Try to repeat them as often as possible. Write your affirmations down on a card or piece of paper and keep it with you so you can refer to them easily.

Start by saying:

I believe in all the affirmations I say to myself and I am fully aware of how they help and heal me.

- I __(your name)__ am full of life and energy.
- I have lots of love in my life.
- I have happiness in my life.
- I am a beautiful person.
- I am a healthy person.
- All my organs work perfectly.
- My body works exactly as it should.
- My body is the perfect weight and height.

- I work out because it will make me strong and healthy.
- My cells breathe in all the oxygen I need.
- My breathing is perfect.
- I am a strong person.
- My muscles are strong and functional.
- I love myself and my body.
- I am the best at what I do.
- My mind is clear and efficient.
- I look in the mirror and see myself as a confident, optimistic and caring person.
- I have faith and believe I can use it to bring me all I need.
- My life is as it should be.
- I am grateful to live and have the power to make my life more positive.
- I can overcome any obstacle.
- I can handle any stress that comes my way.
- I know how to be calm and relaxed.
- I am always improving.
- I am always getting better.
- I can change for the better.

- I love my life.
- I can conquer all that I want to.
- I am a great leader.
- People are always nice to me.
- My parents love me.
- I love my parents.
- I forgive all and I forgive myself.
- I leave the past behind with experiences I learn from.
- I live in the moment.
- I look forward to a wonderful future.
- I will always remain positive.
- I see my life as a wonderful learning experience.
- I am grateful for all I have and continue to receive.
- My mind and thoughts are positive and will make these affirmations true for me.

105

Meditation.

Below is an example of a simple meditation to start with:

- Get into a comfortable position in a chair or lying down. Close your eyes. Place your hands just above your belly button, under your ribs.
- Take in a slow, deep breath through your nose and feel your rib cage expand. Release the breath and repeat, relaxing a bit more every time you exhale.
- Let any thoughts go in and out of your mind.
- Think of a place where you feel safe and comfortable.
- Allow yourself to go to that safe place as you breathe in and out.
- Imagine yourself relaxing in this serene, wonderful place. Let go of any negative thoughts, seeing them literally come out of your body and replace them with positive ones.

- Breathe in and out a few more times.

Take at least 2 minutes to do this when you begin. Go as long as you need and you will be practicing meditation! Start small with a few minutes and build up. Dedicating even 2 minutes a day on a regular basis can make a big difference in your life.

Conclusion

In nurturing your mind, a healthy body and eating right, you allow yourself to open up to a wonderful new world of fun and opportunity.

As the saying goes, if you want to be successful, you have to act, feel and look every bit as successful as you want to be. These days, financial status is not the only yardstick used to measure success.

Incorporate these tips, tricks and pointers into your lifestyle. While it may take a while to adjust and transition into a number of changes, investing in good health will give you the highest return.

Stay In Touch,

Marguerite

Info@BeachChairFitness.com

800-738-9464

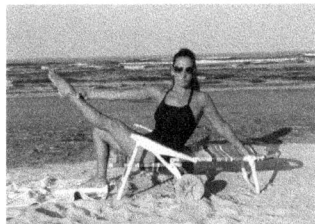

Here is a list of Kindle books by other authors that I think you'll love.

Check them out!

The Diet Dropout's Guide to Natural Weight Loss: Find Your Easiest Path to Naturally Thin by **Stan Spencer**

Weight Loss Boss: How to Finally Win at Losing-- and Take Charge in an Out-of-Control Food World by **David Kirchhoff**

Running SUCKS! How to Run for Fast Weight Loss - For Busy Women Who HATE Running by **Jennifer Jolan**

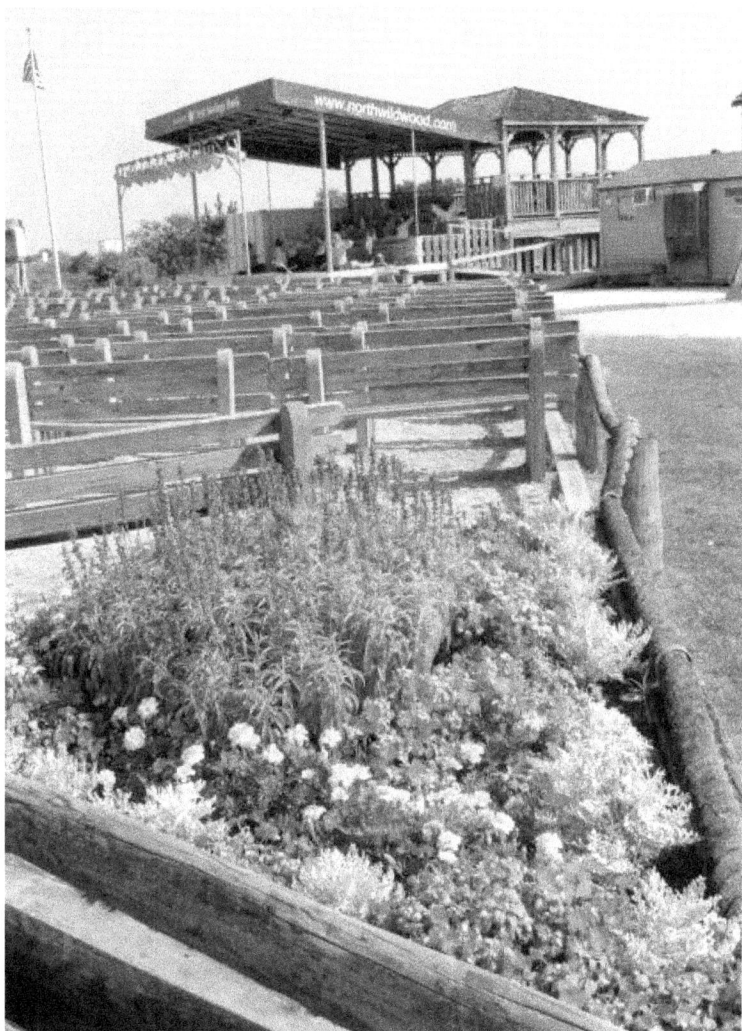

Yoga by the Beach

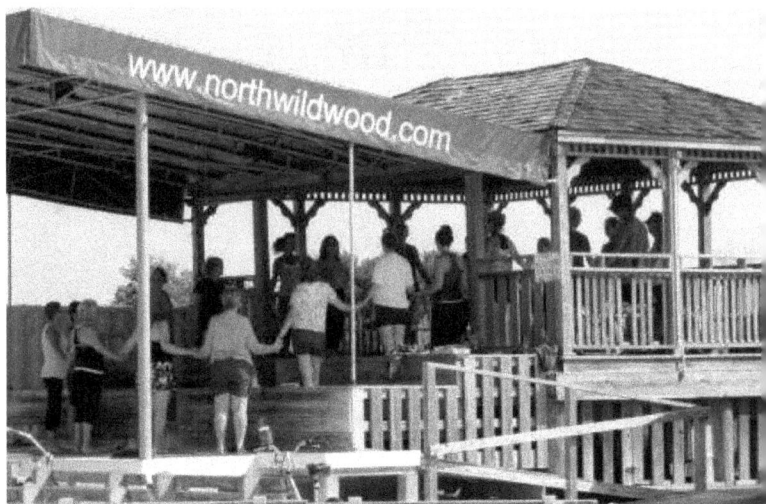

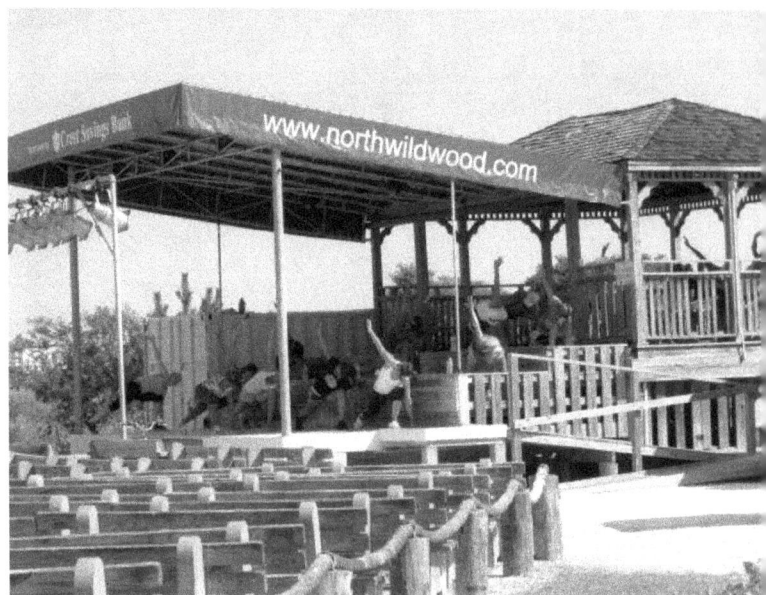

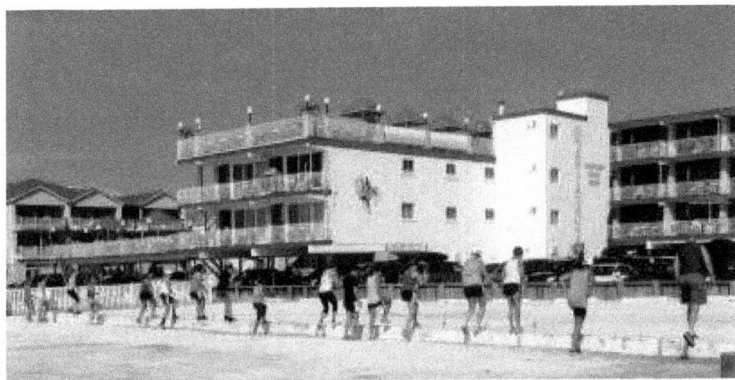

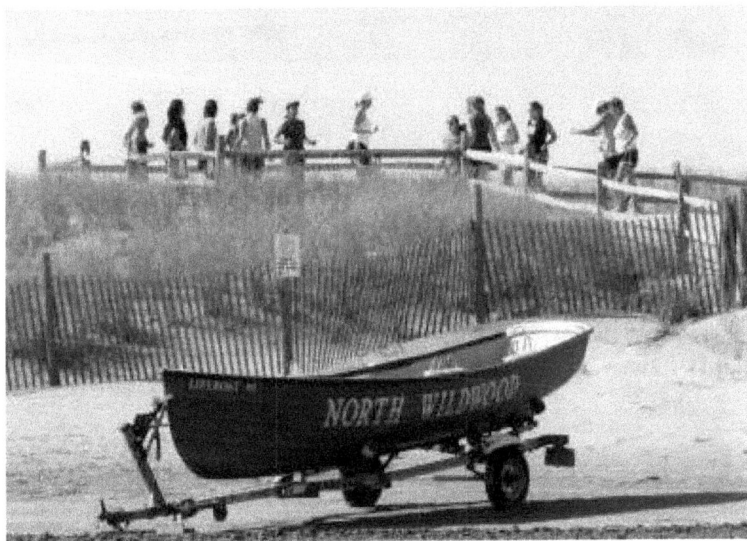

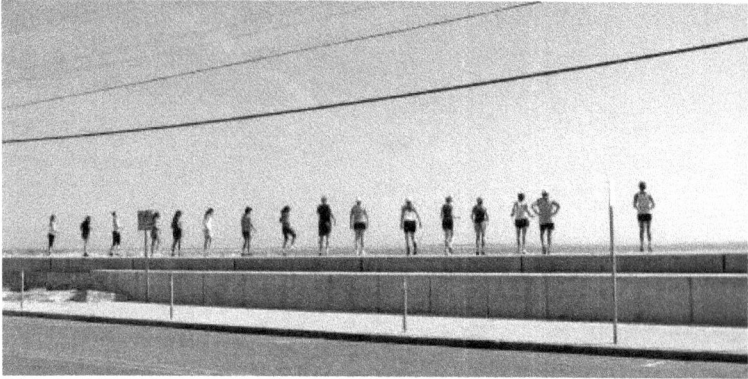

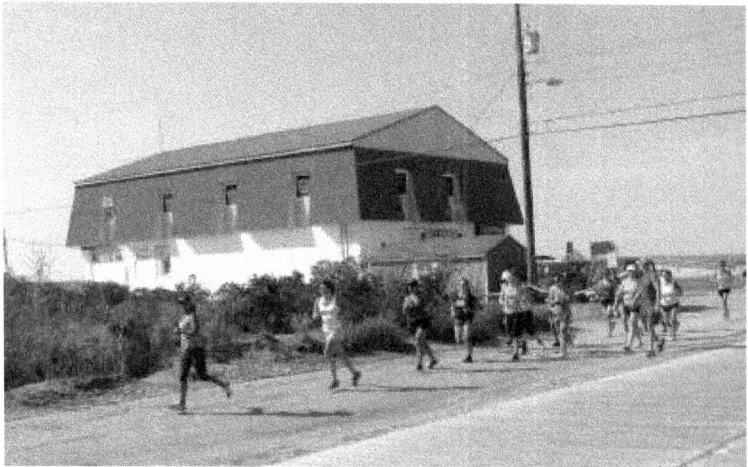

Boot Camp in North Wildwood

www.ingramcontent.com/pod-product-compliance
Lightning Source LLC
Chambersburg PA
CBHW071139280326
41935CB00010B/1295